PRAISE FOR *LIMITLESS*

"In the pivotal section 'Understanding and Integrating Primitive Reflexes,' Dr. Josh Madsen unlocks the mysteries of automatic infant movements that are essential for survival but problematic when retained. With clarity and insight, he reveals how these reflexes can obstruct a child's neurological and developmental progress, impacting their ability to learn and grow. This section doesn't just explain the science—it provides practical steps and engaging activities to help parents and professionals effectively assess and integrate these reflexes. Discover transformative techniques that pave the way for enhanced learning, better coordination, and emotional balance, allowing every child to live a life without limits. An indispensable guide for anyone dedicated to fostering the full potential of the next generation."

—DR. CONNER F. BOR, D.C., DACNB

"Taking our son to see Dr. Josh was one of the best decisions we ever made! Our son has a formal diagnosis of Autism Spectrum Disorder. But we knew we wanted to help him thrive! Dr. Josh has been amazing. He treated Titus' imbalances with supplements and then started adjustments, exercises, and low-level light therapy. A year later he has made huge leaps and bounds and is finally starting to talk to us at 5 years old!"

—JESSICA

"This was the best appointment we have ever had! We have waited for years to have a positive experience like this for our child and we can't wait to continue working with Dr Josh to help improve her health!"

—TRACY

"We are so blessed to have found Infinity. They have changed our daughter's entire life. We could not be more thankful for them and will continue to return as often as we are able. We have worked with almost all of their current staff there. Every single one is top-notch and highly educated in what they are doing! We recommend them over and over!"

—SAMANTHA

"We love Infinity! All three of our boys receive adjustments and therapies from Dr. Josh. Our youngest, who has seen the greatest improvements, struggled with sensory processing and always seemed out of sync. We struggled to know what to do for him until we learned about Dr. Josh. Before therapy, our son struggled to go to stores, parades, even church services because of his extreme sensory issues and consequent behaviors. Now we can go places without major issues. Our youngest can now sit still and quietly in church, as well as focus on age appropriate tasks without melting down. We have also seen great improvement in all three of our children's eye tracking, as well as their vision. We recently had their eyes checked for new glasses and were amazed that their vision had improved immensely! Also, our middle son who struggled to keep up with his peers academically now reads at grade level. We are so thankful for Dr. Josh and his knowledge and skill set to help our sons succeed! Thanks!"

—CASSIE

"THE.MOST.THOROUGH.EVALUATION.MY.CHILD.HAS. EVER.HAD. VERY happy with my daughter's results here. We came for a week intensive to integrate primitive reflexes and help her over-all brain connectivity. They are a very caring office that welcomed my daughter with open arms. I feel they engaged my child appropriately at her level and kept the therapy activities fun."

—BRIANA

"Dr. Josh's book is a step by step recipe book to understand and support neurodivergent children in a core level. I HIGHLY recommend this book!"

—JOOWHYE NAM, D.C.

"Dr. Josh has been amazing in helping me get through my sudden onset of POTS. After working with him for 3 months I'm able to walk, work, and play sports again without my heart rate spiraling out of control. It's been a true blessing, I highly recommend anyone with POTS to go see how he can help."

—CHRISTIAN

"Loved working with Dr. Josh! He's was encouraging, kind, honest and wanted to see my son get better as much as we did. The staff is wonderful and kind. So thankful for his knowledge and gentle approach. HIGHLY recommend!"

—JESSIE

"[Dr. Josh] Explains things so I can understand. There have been amazing improvements in my daughter's coordination."

—WILLIE

"This book is a fantastic resource for practitioners and parents alike! While this book is extremely informative it is also very easy to read and understand. The information provided is extremely valuable for any parent or therapist wanting to help children with many differing challenges."

—ERINN ASKIN, MA OTR/L

"Dr. Josh and his team are phenomenal. They have blessed us with their knowledge and kindness. We are forever grateful."

—GLEN

"Dr. Josh, Laryssa, and the entire Infinity team are not only loving and serving people, but they absolutely are amazing at what they do! My family is so thankful for the cranial and reflex work Dr. Josh continues to provide for our son. He helped him to crawl! With a son who has a complicated medical background, it is hard to know who to trust. Dr. Josh made it an easy decision for our family to place our trust in this office. I encourage anyone who has children (with or without complicated backgrounds) to get their child checked at Infinity Chiropractic. This is one decision that is not optional; it is a necessity for our son's health. Thanks for everything you guys do!"

—ARIANN

"Dr. Josh and his entire staff are no doubt the best! From the second you walk in the front door you are greeted with smiles and the most helpful people. Then you are met with professionals who listen to every and all concerns. They are great with patients of all ages. We will always be so thankful for the staff that has been a part of our son's journey."

—ACACIA

"We started going to Infinity 5-6 months ago. My son (7 years old) had multiple developmental delays including gross motor, fine motor, speech, and vision. We have spent many hours doing PT, OT, Speech Therapy, and Vision Therapy, and therapists have always said the same thing "He is making progress but much slower than I would expect." So, I decided to go to Infinity. One of my top concerns was his vision, I knew it was affecting him in school, and vision therapy hadn't helped. We worked through primitive reflexes and worked on his vision, and it has improved! My son says he now only sees one set of words on the page. In February they tested his reading and he was reading 35 WPM. They just tested him in early May and he tested 70 WPM. He doubled his speed in 3 months. His balance is also much improved, and his handwriting is improving."

—EMILY

"Very knowledgeable and caring doctors and staff. Life-changing experience for my daughter! We are so thankful for this clinic"

—KIMBERLY

"Our 13-year-old son came to see Dr. Josh with diagnoses of dyslexia, ADHD, and slow information processing. At his first appointment, we learned he still retained 3 primitive reflexes, had very poor development of his vestibular system, and had several eye-tracking issues. We'd never known he had double vision up close and trouble tracking and converging his eyes! After three months of chiropractic care, prescribed exercise program, and eye strengthening exercises, the primitive reflexes are no longer interfering with learning and attention. We've seen amazing improvement in his vestibular development and eye tracking. We continue exercises at home for those. I have been in tears many times when home-schooling him and seeing how much more smoothly his brain is working! Integrating new information and recalling previously learned information is where I see the biggest positive change for him. We look forward to his continuing improvement! I wish we had known about this when our son was first learning to read and we could've avoided years of frustration for him. Thank you so much, Dr. Josh and team!!!"

—TINA

"At first I thought Infinity was promising more than it could deliver on for our son. Then over time, we saw significant improvement in his coordination and strength.

Today, he can do things he wasn't even close to doing 8 months ago. He's hitting baseballs and climbing warped walls, and his confidence is soaring. Thanks Infinity!"

—BRANDON

"I don't even know where to start on how much Dr. Josh has helped our 2 boys. We had been doing a different type of reflex integration on our oldest son for close to 3 1/2 years with very little progress. We were struggling to keep him going to his appointments, and he was getting discouraged because he knew he wasn't making much progress. He has debilitating anxiety levels, poor sleep habits, and a very selective diet due to sensory issues - he has been stuck in fight or flight for as long as we can remember. We always thought that he needed some type of supplements but he refused any type of over-the-counter supplement, and when we would have lab work, we couldn't pinpoint what nutrients he was lacking. Our youngest son has outbursts on a regular basis and at times can be very aggressive. He is averse to touch and was struggling to interact appropriately with his peers in school. I was referred to Dr. Josh and our lives have changed drastically over the course of a little over a month. We started by cutting gluten out of both kids' diets (something that had never been mentioned to us by all the doctors we had been in touch with). We then did another test to see what supplements would help our oldest. We've seen huge improvements in his mood, energy levels, and confidence. In the short time we've been seeing Dr. Josh, all of my oldest son's reflexes are now gone and our youngest boy is well on his way. During the holidays I had several family members comment on the difference they've seen in our boys. They didn't struggle with sensory overload at the family functions the way they previously had and socialized on a level we've never seen them do before. The boys absolutely LOVE to see Dr. Josh, and he has been a miracle worker for our family. My son even asked me why we didn't come to Dr. Josh 3 years ago. :) I can't recommend Dr. Josh enough!!!!!!"

—KELLEY

"Dr. Josh and his team are fantastic!! They are all so kind and personable. I appreciate their holistic approach, and we have seen great improvements in digestion, behavior, and speech!"

—JENNIFER

LIMITLESS

LIMITLESS

Integrate Primitive Reflexes and
Transform Your Child's Ability
to Read, Learn, and Live

Dr. Josh Madsen, D.C.

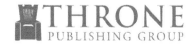
THRONE
PUBLISHING GROUP

I dedicate this book to my supportive family and to my loving wife and son who have inspired me to help as many kids as I can.

TABLE OF CONTENTS

FOREWORD

t is with immense pleasure and honor that I write this foreword for Dr. Josh Madsen's groundbreaking book, a vital resource for parents, educators, and healthcare professionals alike. Having known Josh for over a decade since our graduate school days, I have witnessed firsthand his deep commitment and relentless pursuit of understanding and addressing neurodevelopmental challenges in children.

Dr. Madsen's expertise is not just rooted in his impressive academic background. His real-world impact is evident in the hundreds, if not thousands, of children whose lives he has transformed. Through his work, Josh has documented significant improvements in children's abilities, capturing not only their advancements, but also the profound emotional relief and joy of their families.

This book emerges from Dr. Madsen's extensive clinical experience and personal journey, both of which have shaped his unique perspective on pediatric neurodevelopment. Unlike traditional approaches that often compartmentalize symptoms, Josh's methodology is holistic, addressing the foundational neurological systems that underpin a child's ability to learn and thrive.

In "Limitless" Dr. Madsen offers more than just insights; he provides a pathway to hope and healing. He artfully illustrates how seemingly unrelated physical activities, like addressing primitive reflexes and enhancing motor development, can dramatically improve cognitive functions, including reading and learning. The book meticulously guides readers through understanding how developmental systems support learning, identifying signs of delays, and applying effective interventions.

What sets this book apart is its threefold purpose: to educate, to guide, and to empower. It is structured to not only impart knowledge, but also to equip you with practical tools to assess and aid your child's development. Dr. Madsen's narrative is compelling, weaving scientific evidence with personal anecdotes that resonate with anyone who has witnessed a child struggle to fit the conventional molds of learning.

By the end of this book, you will not only grasp the crucial role of primitive reflexes in your child's development but also have at your disposal actionable steps to foster their growth toward a life without limits. Dr. Madsen's message is clear and potent—a life of boundless potential awaits, and the journey begins with understanding and action.

As you turn the pages, prepare to be inspired and transformed. Join Dr. Madsen in making a profound difference in the lives of our children, helping them navigate their unique paths with confidence and resilience. This book is more than an educational tool; it is a beacon of hope and a testament to what can be achieved when we view challenges as opportunities for growth and learning.

Your journey to a deeper understanding and practical application of how to support your child's development starts here. Dive in with an open heart and mind, ready to embark on an enlightening path that promises to enrich your perspective and equip you with the knowledge to create a brighter future for your child. I promise, you will not regret it.

Dr. Trevor Eason

INTRODUCTION

I t is quite remarkable to improve a child's reading skills without focusing solely on reading itself. After working with thousands of kids, I have witnessed this phenomenon repeatedly, seeing children make leaps of entire grade levels in reading within just a few months. I'm not talking about progressing from one letter to another in the reading system used in schools; I'm talking about going from the reading level expected at the start of third grade to the level expected at the end of fourth grade. Astonishingly, this progress was achieved without directly working on the child's reading skills. Instead, it was accomplished by developing the foundational systems necessary for reading, learning, and living without limits.

It is incredible to think that the development required for the aforementioned scenario primarily occurs through motor and movement development, but it's true. Neurodevelopmental delays are most often caused by a nervous system that hasn't yet properly and systematically matured. We can help it mature and therefore facilitate reading, learning, and overall life skills by eliminating various developmental reflexes and enhancing a child's balance and eye-tracking abilities.

The purposes of this book are threefold. First, I want to educate readers on the importance of developing these neurological and developmental systems to support efficient learning. Second, I want to share how to identify if such systems may be delayed in your child. Finally, I want to talk about intensives, which I've found to be the fastest and most effective intervention for developing such systems in children who are lagging behind.

Through this book I aim to offer you a concise overview of primitive reflexes, focusing on those most crucial for learning. This book will provide you with quick and actionable tasks to perform with your child to determine if these reflexes are present. If they are, I have provided additional steps for you to follow at the end of the book.

By the time you read the final page, you will understand the impact that retained primitive reflexes can have on your child's learning. You will also have a set of practical tips and tools to help your child overcome these challenges and improve their learning and living experiences. I hope this book blesses you with the knowledge and tools to assist your child, just as I was blessed when I first learned about these developmental reflexes. A life without limits for you and your child is just around the corner.

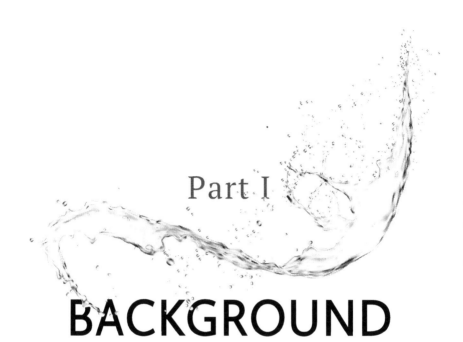

Part I

BACKGROUND

CONNECTION OR COINCIDENCE?

I vividly recall a child with learning difficulties who came to me early in my practice. I had no idea then that the work I was about to undertake could help numerous struggling readers and learners. I conducted an examination and discovered the presence of primitive reflexes, so I began working with the child to integrate these reflexes. While chiropractic care was also part of the treatment, our primary focus was addressing primitive reflexes.

The child had an asymmetrical tonic neck reflex (ATNR), which typically disappears around six months of age, before crawling begins. Additionally, they had a symmetrical tonic neck reflex (STNR), which should dissipate after eight months. From their history, it became evident that the child had never army crawled. They experienced difficulties with hands and knees crawling but started walking at around nine or ten months, which is earlier than the expected twelve months. Contrary to popular belief, walking early is not a sign of superior development but rather of abnormal reflex development.

As we worked on eliminating the child's primitive reflexes, something remarkable occurred. Their learning abilities improved dramatically, and within a few months they made a significant leap of an entire grade level. This may sound unbelievable, but such outcomes are quite typical in our office. In this case, the child was in fourth grade and progressed from a third-grade reading level to the end of the fourth-grade level in just three months.

At that time, I had no idea that addressing primitive reflexes could bring such transformative changes. I thought it might have been a mere coincidence, unaware that such profound changes were even possible. However, the patient's mother shared the story with a friend who also had a child struggling with reading, and I ended up treating that child as well with similar positive results. Subsequently, another child was referred by their teacher, again with comparable outcomes. Even the optometrist of one of these children noticed the change and started referring numerous children with reading issues to me.

The pattern continued, and I can now confidently say that approximately 90% of children with learning difficulties experience significant improvement through the methods discussed in this book. The astonishing aspect is that they witness substantial changes in their reading abilities during our program without prior knowledge. This highlights the importance of motor development in laying the foundation for learning and reading. The fundamental premise of this program revolves around three key points:

- Addressing primitive reflexes
- Developing balance centers
- Enhancing eye-tracking abilities

These three deficits are commonly observed in nearly every child with learning disabilities. From a developmental perspective, these systems form the foundation for normal brain function and efficient learning.

PYRAMID OF DEVELOPMENT and LEARNING

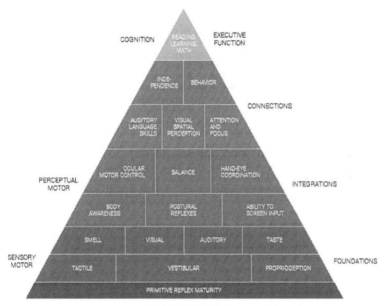

I also typically find these deficits in children diagnosed with dyslexia. It is important to note that while these deficits are often present in such children, they do not necessarily cause dyslexia and are often distinct issues. Nonetheless, these foundational deficits play a role in the child's learning difficulties. Extensive research supports the existence of these deficits in children with dyslexia.

CONNECTING THE DOTS

I struggled initially to comprehend the connection between working on primitive reflexes and the subsequent improvement in learning. However, as I delved deeper into research, I discovered substantial evidence supporting the link between motor development, cognition, and executive functioning skills. Furthermore, extensive evidence supports the associations among primitive reflexes, balance center development, ocular center development, and learning.

Have you ever heard someone mention the connection between a lack of normal crawling and reading difficulties later in life? Well, it turns out that statement is true. The development that takes place in the first year of life is crucial for supporting proper future brain development. These early motor milestones hold great importance and are sometimes missed in almost all children with learning issues.

Take a moment to reflect on your child's history. If you answer "no" to any of these questions, it is likely a contributing factor to your child's learning struggles.

1. Did your child engage in army crawling at five to seven months?

2. Did your child crawl on hands and knees (cross crawl) at six to eight months?
3. Did your child start walking at eleven-and-a-half to twelve-and-a-half months?
4. Does your child demonstrate good posture?
5. Did your child learn to tie their shoes at an appropriate age?
6. Did your child learn to ride a bicycle at an appropriate age?
7. Did your child exhibit coordination similar to other children as they grew up?
8. Does your child run symmetrically and with good coordination?

The systems we develop in the first year of life form the foundation for motor development, which is essential for cognitive center development. Therefore, if you answered "no" to any of these questions because your child did not achieve these milestones or did not achieve them within the expected time frames, it indicates a lack of appropriate motor system development, which could mean lack of cognitive development, executive functioning skills, and subsequent learning difficulties.

WALKING IN THEIR SHOES

Imagine your precious child sitting anxiously in their classroom, praying not to be picked to read out loud. They're all too aware that if they're chosen, their peers might discover their struggles and tease them. Picture them looking over to their classmates during a test—not because they want to cheat, but simply because they can't read the questions as swiftly as others do. They're terrified of standing out, of being seen as slow or less intelligent.

When they look at a book, their eyes constantly shifting and adjusting, the words seem to dance around the page. Even though they know each word and understand its meanings, the constantly moving text makes it difficult to keep up. Imagine them trying to copy from a chalkboard but falling behind because their eyes take longer to focus on the words. In the process, they miss the teacher's explanations because they're so busy trying to jot down a few words. Despite these challenges, they do their best to blend in, to avoid feeling different or needing special assistance. It's a testament to their intelligence and resilience that they've managed to get by in this way for so long.

This was my own experience in school, and you can see why it wasn't a time I fondly remember. For many years, I believed I was less capable, and I was unable to comprehend why school seemed so straightforward and enjoyable for other kids. Despite working tirelessly with tutors and my dedicated parents, my academic performance never reflected my effort. It wasn't until I addressed some underdeveloped foundational skills such as eliminating retained primitive reflexes, working on my eyesight, and adjusting my diet that my grades improved dramatically. I went from average grades to straight As and even made the dean's list when I figured all this out in college. I've come to believe that this struggle was a lesson in disguise—a blessing from above rather than a curse. It equipped me with the understanding and empathy to help children who face similar struggles. Knowing that many parents are desperate for that same understanding and empathy, let's delve into Part II: Primitive Reflexes.

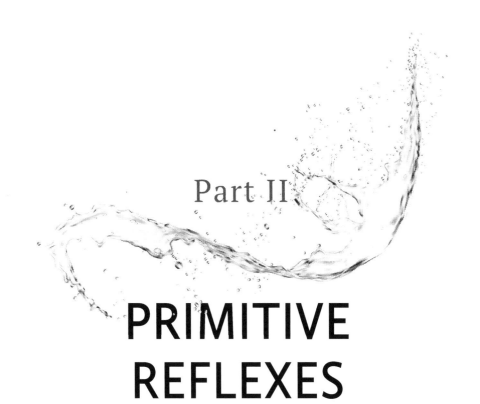

Part II

PRIMITIVE
REFLEXES

PRIMITIVE REFLEXES DEFINED

Primitive reflexes, also known as infantile reflexes or neonatal reflexes, are a set of automatic movements and responses in newborns that typically disappear within the first few months of life as the infant's nervous system matures. If the infant's nervous system is not developing appropriately, these reflexes will last longer than they should.

The brainstem, the spinal cord, and multiple different areas of the higher cortex mediate these reflexes. From a developmental perspective, they serve as the building blocks of all brain development. Therefore, if they do not mature properly, the rest of the brain cannot efficiently develop either. They are typically responses to a specific stimulus such as touch or movement, and they result in a specific movement or response.

One example is the Moro reflex, which is elicited by sudden changes in position or loud noises and results in the infant extending their arms and legs before bringing them back in close to the body. Another example is the rooting reflex, which is elicited by touching the infant's cheek and results in the infant turning their head toward the stimulus.

Primitive reflexes are considered a normal part of infant development and important for survival and early motor development.

This is important because there are many studies on early motor development and later learning skills. These studies have concluded that the better the early motor development, the better the child's early learning performance. However, the persistence of basic reflexes past the average age at which they typically disappear may indicate underlying neurological or developmental problems and call for further evaluation.

PRIMITIVE REFLEXES, DEVELOPMENT, AND LEARNING

Primitive reflexes are important for the survival and early motor development of infants. However, if these reflexes continue after the average age at which they typically disappear, they may have a variety of negative effects on development and learning. Here's a simplified explanation of how retained primitive reflexes affect learning and reading:

1. Motor skills: Retained primitive reflexes can interfere with the development of postural reflexes, which are necessary for controlling body position, movement, and balance. This can lead to difficulties with gross and fine motor skills, both of which are important for writing, holding a pencil, and coordinating the eye movements needed for reading.

2. Eye tracking and coordination: Many primitive reflexes involve eye movements. If these reflexes are retained, they can interfere with the ability to control eye movements. This can lead to difficulties with skills such as tracking a line of text in a book or copying from a chalkboard.

3. Focus and attention: Retained primitive reflexes can cause a child to be in a constant state of alert, making it difficult

for them to relax, focus, or pay attention in class. This can affect their ability to concentrate on tasks such as reading and writing.

4. Spatial awareness and perception: Some primitive reflexes are involved in the development of spatial awareness and perception. If these reflexes are retained, a child may struggle with understanding the relationship between themselves and the space around them, which can affect their ability to process visual information and lead to reading and writing difficulties.

5. Sensory integration: Primitive reflexes help with the process of integrating sensory information. If these reflexes are retained, it can lead to sensory processing issues, which can affect a child's ability to manage and respond to the sensory information involved in classroom learning.

It is important to note that there are over thirty primitive reflexes that can contribute to all of the systems mentioned above to develop. I'll concentrate on the most significant ones relating to reading and learning that I've discovered to be true in clinical practice and my own research. When you concentrate on the reflexes I discuss in this book, you will often see massive changes in learning and development.

COMMON PRIMITIVE REFLEXES

Several primitive reflexes commonly exist in newborns and usually disappear within the first few months of life as the nervous system matures. Here's an overview of some of the most common primitive reflexes, along with some typical symptoms observed when these reflexes persist.

It's important to note that not every child will exhibit all symptoms because these reflexes can be present at varying degrees.

1. Moro reflex
    *   Startling easily in response to loud noises, bright lights, or sudden movements
    *   Difficulty with balance and coordination
    *   Anxiety and emotional sensitivity
    *   Difficulty adapting to new situations or environments

2. Asymmetrical tonic neck reflex (ATNR)
    *   Difficulty with eye tracking and visual focus, which can affect reading
    *   Challenges with hand–eye coordination, affecting writing and other fine motor tasks

- Trouble crossing the midline of the body, affecting activities such as playing sports

3. Symmetrical tonic neck reflex (STNR)
   - Poor posture, especially when sitting or crawling
   - Difficulty with balance and coordination
   - Challenges with visual focus, particularly when looking from near to far (or vice versa)
   - Trouble with hand–eye coordination and fine motor skills

4. Tonic labyrinthine reflex (TLR)
   - Issues with balance and coordination, affecting activities such as riding a bike or playing sports
   - Poor muscle tone, either too stiff (hypertonic) or too floppy (hypotonic)
   - Difficulty with spatial awareness and navigating the environment
   - Trouble maintaining a proper head position when reading or writing

5. Palmar grasp reflex
   - Involuntary grasping of objects placed in the hand, making it difficult to let go
   - Difficulty with fine motor skills such as writing, buttoning clothes, or using utensils
   - Potential challenges with hand–eye coordination

6. Plantar grasp reflex
   - Involuntary curling of the toes when the sole of the foot is touched

- Difficulty with balance and walking, especially on uneven surfaces
- Challenges when learning to wear shoes or transitioning between different types of footwear

7. Spinal Galant reflex
   - Involuntary hip movement when the lower back is stroked on one side
   - Fidgeting or squirming when sitting for extended periods, which may affect attention and focus
   - Bed-wetting or issues with bladder control
   - Difficulty with balance and coordination

8. Rooting reflex
   - Turning the head and opening the mouth in response to a touch on the cheek
   - Essential for breastfeeding, but its persistence could indicate issues with oral motor development
   - Potential challenges with speech and language development

9. Sucking reflex
   - Involuntary sucking when an object is placed in the mouth
   - If not properly integrated, may indicate difficulties with oral motor development or feeding
   - Potential challenges with speech and language development

We assess these reflexes by grading them on a scale of 0 to 4. A score of 4 indicates a fully present and strong reflex, whereas a score of 0 suggests the reflex is not present at all. For example, a child may exhibit a Moro reflex graded at 4, presenting many of the associated symptoms. Conversely, the same child could display an ATNR graded at 2, demonstrating only a few or potentially none of the corresponding symptoms.

However, the presence of any un-integrated reflex, regardless of its degree or associated symptoms, needs to be addressed to ensure comprehensive rehabilitation. Every reflex plays a crucial role in a child's development, and our goal is to ensure all reflexes are appropriately integrated for a well-functioning and developing child.

It's important to note that the presence of one or more of these behaviors does not automatically indicate a retained reflex. An evaluation is necessary to determine if a reflex is retained and if it is contributing to a child's developmental challenges. For the purposes of this book, I'll discuss the ATNR, STNR, and TLR in detail because they are the most common reflexes found in reading-impaired children.

Asymmetrical Tonic Neck Reflex

The ATNR is a primitive reflex that is typically present in newborns and disappears around four to six months. This reflex is elicited by turning the infant's head to one side, resulting in the extension of the arm and leg on the same side as the head that is turned and the flexion of the arm and leg on the opposite side.

The ATNR plays an important role in the development of the infant's motor and sensory systems. It helps establish connections among the visual, vestibular, and motor systems and is thought to be important for the development of hand–eye coordination, head control, and the ability to reach for and manipulate objects.

However, if the ATNR persists beyond the average age they should disappear, it can interfere with the development of these skills. For example, it can interfere with an infant's ability to visually track objects and can cause difficulties with hand–eye coordination and reaching. A persistent ATNR can also cause an infant to develop asymmetrically because one side of the body is more active than the other. Persistent ATNR can also lead to difficulties with attention and learning; the reflex can interfere with an infant's ability to focus on visual and auditory stimuli because they may be distracted by the involuntary movement of their arms and legs.

We often see the ATNR leading to impaired eye tracking, particularly when moving from side to side. It's common to observe substantial skips and jumps in a child's eyes as they attempt to follow an object. This could result in the eyes making sudden movements during reading, causing the child to lose their place or struggle with tracking a line of text.

In summary, while the ATNR is an important reflex for the development of the infant's motor and sensory systems, the persistence of the reflex beyond the average age at which it should disappear can interfere with the development of skills such as hand–eye coordination, attention, and reading. Below is a link to my reflex assessment of a patient so you can see what a positive reflex looks like. Test this on your child to see if it is present.

Here is a link with information about assessing the ATNR: https://youtu.be/aYDVuyqf9aE.

Symmetrical Tonic Neck Reflex

The STNR is a primitive reflex that emerges around six to nine months of age and typically disappears around nine to eleven months.

The reflex is elicited by changes in the position of the infant's head relative to their body, resulting in a change in the position of their arms and legs.

The STNR has two phases: the flexor phase and the extensor phase. In the flexor phase, when the infant's head is flexed (i.e., chin to chest), their arms bend and their legs straighten. In the extensor phase, when the infant's head is extended (i.e., looking up), their arms will straighten and their legs will bend.

The STNR plays an important role in the development of the infant's motor and sensory systems. It helps establish connections between the visual, vestibular, and motor systems and is thought to be important for the development of crawling and creeping as well as other forms of locomotion. However, if the STNR persists beyond the average age at which it should disappear, it can interfere with the development of these skills. For example, it can make it difficult for the infant to coordinate the movements of their arms and legs, which can interfere in turn with crawling and other forms of locomotion.

Persistent STNR can also affect the infant's ability to sit upright and maintain good posture because the reflex can cause the infant's legs to straighten when their head is extended, which can make it difficult to balance and maintain a stable sitting position. We often see this create a scenario where the child is constantly moving or fidgeting, which is distracting for a child who is learning.

This reflex is also found in children with an eye condition called convergence insufficiency, which is when your eyes are unable to work together when looking at nearby objects. This condition causes one eye to turn outward instead of inward with the other eye, creating double or blurred vision.

Symptoms of convergence insufficiency can include the following:

1. Eye strain or fatigue: the eyes tire quickly or feel uncomfortable, especially during close work such as reading or computer use
2. Headaches: frequent or recurring, often after reading or doing other close work
3. Double vision: seeing two images of a single object
4. Difficulty reading: trouble reading or slow reading, losing place, or finding words jumping around on the page
5. Difficulty concentrating: finding it hard to concentrate when reading or doing other close work
6. Blurred vision: vision might be blurry at near distances, or may have difficulty changing focus between near and far objects
7. Squinting or closing one eye: squinting or closing one eye to see better
8. Dizziness or motion sickness: feeling unsteady or having a sense of movement or spinning

Here is a link with information about assessing the STNR: https://youtu.be/xpnTKTYP95M

Tonic Labyrinthine Reflex

The TLR is a primitive reflex that is present at birth and typically disappears around six months. The reflex is elicited by changes in the position of the infant's head relative to their body, resulting in changes in their muscle tone and posture.

The TLR has two phases: the flexor phase and the extensor phase. In the flexor phase, when the infant is placed in a supine position (lying on their back), their arms and legs will flex (bend), and their head will extend (tilt back). In the extensor phase, when the infant is placed in a prone position (lying on their stomach), their arms and legs will extend (straighten), and their head will flex (tilt forward).

The TLR plays an important role in the development of the infant's motor and sensory systems. It helps establish the connections among the visual, vestibular, and motor systems and is thought to be important for developing posture, balance, and coordination.

However, if the TLR persists beyond the average age at which it should disappear, it can interfere with development of these skills. For example, it can make it difficult for the infant to maintain a stable sitting position because their head may tilt back when in a supine position or tilt forward when in a prone position. It can also interfere with the development of crawling and other forms of locomotion by making it difficult to coordinate movements of the arms and legs.

Persistent TLR can also affect the infant's ability to process sensory information, causing them to be overly sensitive to changes in their position or to become disoriented when placed in different positions.

Regarding learning, the TLR can interfere with the development of more complex skills and reflexes necessary for efficient learning. Here are some ways a retained TLR could potentially affect reading and learning:

1. Gross and fine motor skills: TLR is closely related to the development of gross and fine motor skills. If TLR is retained, it can lead to poor muscle tone and coordination, which can affect handwriting, the ability to sit still, and overall physical coordination.
2. Visual tracking and eye movements: TLR also plays a role in the development of certain eye movements. If the reflex

is retained, a child may struggle with visual tracking, which is important for reading. They might find it hard to follow a line of text without losing their place.

3. Spatial awareness and balance: A retained TLR can affect a child's balance and spatial awareness, leading to potential difficulties in sports and activities that require coordination. Additionally, problems with spatial awareness can affect mathematical skills and understanding of spatial concepts in reading and writing.

4. Concentration and attention: Children with a retained TLR might find it hard to stay still and concentrate, which can affect their ability to focus during classroom activities, including reading and writing.

5. Sequencing and organization skills: TLR influences the ability to understand sequences and organize thoughts, both crucial for complex learning tasks. If this reflex is retained, a child may struggle with tasks that require sequencing such as spelling, writing, and reading comprehension.

Here is a link with information about assessing the TLR: https://youtu.be/YDvjLI8eU7M.

Other primitive reflexes that can affect development and learning include the palmar reflex, plantar reflex, and Babinski reflex. The palmar reflex causes a child to involuntarily grasp an object placed in their hand, which can interfere with the development of fine motor skills. The plantar reflex causes the toes to curl when the sole of the foot is stimulated, which can interfere with balance and coordination. The Babinski reflex causes the big toe to extend when the sole of the foot is stimulated, which can interfere with walking and other gross motor skills.

Overall, the impact of retained primitive reflexes on development and learning can vary depending on the individual child and the specific reflex involved. However, addressing retained primitive reflexes through exercises and therapies can help improve a child's motor skills, sensory processing, and overall development.

PURPOSE OF PRIMITIVE REFLEXES

Primitive reflexes serve an important function in the early stages of human development. They are automatic, innate movements and responses present in newborns that help them survive and adapt to their environment. For example, the rooting reflex is elicited by touch to the infant's cheek and results in the infant turning their head toward the stimulus, which helps them find and suck on a nipple for nourishment.

These reflexes also play a role in the development of the nervous system and motor skills. They help establish connections between the sensory and motor systems, which are important for the development of more sophisticated movements and abilities such as reaching and grasping. For example, the palmar reflex helps infants to hold objects and develop their hand strength, which is important for their ability to manipulate objects and explore their environment.

However, primitive reflexes should disappear within the first few months of life as the nervous system matures and more sophisticated motor and sensory skills develop. The persistence of primitive reflexes beyond the average age at which they should disappear may be indicative of underlying neurological or developmental issues and can affect development and learning in several ways, as described in previous discussions.

INTEGRATION OF PRIMITIVE REFLEXES

Primitive reflexes are the automatic, involuntary movements that are present at birth and gradually disappear as the nervous system matures. As a child develops, these reflexes become integrated into more complex voluntary movements and are eventually replaced by more sophisticated motor patterns.

The integration of primitive reflexes is a crucial part of neuro-development. As the nervous system matures, the brain's control over movement becomes more refined, and voluntary movements accordingly become more coordinated and purposeful. The primitive reflexes that were once necessary for survival such as the sucking and startle reflex gradually lose their dominance over voluntary movements and become less apparent.

The process of integrating primitive reflexes is not automatic and requires proper neurodevelopmental input. When a child experiences proper sensory stimulation such as through play, movement, and social interaction, the brain can integrate primitive reflexes into more complex movements. Conversely, when a child does not receive adequate sensory input or experiences stress or trauma, primitive reflexes may persist or become hyperactive, leading to developmental delays or disorders.

The integration of primitive reflexes is a critical component of the nervous system's maturation. As the brain develops, the primitive reflexes once necessary for survival gradually become integrated into more complex and sophisticated movements, ultimately leading to more coordinated and purposeful movements. I often tell my patients that the brain develops out of movement, and the better that movement is, the better the brain develops.

RETAINED PRIMITIVE REFLEXES

Retained primitive reflexes can significantly affect a child's ability to function optimally. Because these reflexes disappear as the nervous system matures, the persistence of these reflexes beyond the expected age range can indicate a delay or disruption in the normal development of the nervous system. This can happen for a multitude of reasons, including drug exposure in the womb, birth trauma, lack of sensory stimulation in the first months or years of life, infections, head trauma, and even food sensitivities. The key to helping a child integrate their reflexes is often eliminating inflammatory foods from their diet and providing them with appropriate nutrients. According to previous research in this area, the primary approach to addressing these reflexes is through movement exercises. However, in many cases these exercises have been attempted for months or years without success. Often, by simply altering their diet, we witness the integration of their reflexes. This is why I believe that this topic delves much deeper than the simplistic notion of "Do your exercises, and they will disappear."

Retained primitive reflexes can affect many areas of a child's life, including their motor skills, sensory processing, attention and learning, and emotional regulation. For example, the Moro reflex, which is typically present in infants and disappears around four to six months, is associated with the startle response and can lead to increased anxiety and difficulty with self-regulation if it persists.

As this reflex develops, it should go away and turn into a more appropriate, voluntary startle response, but in many children, it doesn't go away appropriately. Instead, the reflex is retained. Whenever the child moves too quickly or if light, sound, or touch is too abrasive, they startle. Their pupils dilate, their heart rate rises, and they go into a fight-or-flight state. Their body's reaction to a minor stimulus would be similar to your response if you were walking down a dim hallway and someone jumped out and scared you. Your body would do the same thing: pupils dilate, heart rate goes up, and you have to decide whether to fight or run.

When children retain this primitive reflex, they're constantly stuck in a fight-or-flight state, generating anxiety and behavioral and attention issues. These children have a hard time transitioning from place to place or task to task because they don't know what's going to startle them next. They often have allergies or asthma because when they're startled, their body releases adrenaline and cortisol, which deregulates the immune system. In the coming pages, I'll show you how to test your child for this reflex. If it is present, you've likely found a major underlying cause of your child being stuck in sympathetic dominance.

Similarly, the ATNR, which is present from birth to six months, can interfere with hand–eye coordination and affect ability to read and write. It can also hinder proper development of our balance centers, resulting in difficulties for children learning to ride a bicycle or engage in activities that rely on well-developed balance systems.

The palmar reflex, which entails grasping objects with the fingers, can pose challenges for individuals in releasing objects and developing fine motor skills. This often leads to issues with handwriting or learning to tie shoes.

In addition to motor and sensory issues, retained primitive reflexes can also affect an individual's emotional and social functioning. For example, the fear paralysis reflex, which involves freezing in response to a perceived threat, can lead to avoidance and social anxiety.

Overall, retained primitive reflexes can significantly affect an individual's overall development and quality of life. It is important to identify and address these reflexes through appropriate interventions.

AREAS OF THE BRAIN ASSOCIATED WITH RETAINED PRIMITIVE REFLEXES

Retained reflexes are linked to immature or underdeveloped neural connections in various regions of the brain. Different primitive reflexes are associated with different areas of the brain because they each serve specific developmental purposes. Here are some brain areas commonly associated with retained primitive reflexes:

1. Brainstem: The brainstem is the most primitive part of the brain and is responsible for many basic life-sustaining functions such as heart rate, breathing, and arousal. Primitive reflexes originate in the brainstem, and their persistence may indicate an issue with the maturation or development of this region.

2. Cerebellum: The cerebellum plays a crucial role in coordinating movement, balance, and muscle tone. Retained reflexes such as the TLR and ATNR, which affect balance and coordination, may suggest a delay in the development of the cerebellum.

3. Basal ganglia: The basal ganglia are involved in the control of voluntary motor movements, procedural learning, and habit formation. Retained reflexes that affect motor control

such as the palmar reflex or STNR may be associated with immature or underdeveloped neural connections in the basal ganglia.

4. Prefrontal cortex: The prefrontal cortex is responsible for higher cognitive functions such as decision-making, problem-solving, and paying attention. Retained reflexes can interfere with the development of these higher-order cognitive skills, indicating issues with the maturation of the prefrontal cortex.

5. Parietal lobe: The parietal lobe processes sensory information and integrates sensory input with motor output. Retained reflexes that affect sensory processing such as the spinal Galant reflex or the rooting reflex, may be associated with delays in the development of the parietal lobe.

6. Occipital lobe: The occipital lobe is primarily responsible for visual processing. Retained reflexes that affect visual functions such as eye tracking or visual focus may be linked to the development of the occipital lobe.

It is essential to note that the brain functions as an interconnected network, and a delay in one area can also affect other areas. Retained reflexes may be associated with broader neural developmental issues, and addressing them through targeted interventions can help improve overall brain function and development.

ASSESSING PRIMITIVE REFLEXES

Assessment tools and techniques used to assess primitive reflexes vary depending on the professional conducting the evaluation. Pediatricians, occupational therapists, functional neurologists, and chiropractors specializing in pediatrics all use different methods to assess primitive reflexes. Here is an overview of some common assessment tools and techniques:

1. Clinical observation: A key component of assessing primitive reflexes is observing a child's behavior, movements, and responses to stimuli. The professional will look for signs of retained reflexes such as difficulty with balance, coordination, or crossing the midline. They may also ask the child to perform specific movements or tasks to evaluate their motor skills and response to different sensory inputs. In our office, we run a child through motor, balance, visual, and visual analysis skills. We then conduct computerized testing for the balance centers and eye tracking centers, allowing us to create standardizations based on age-related peers to determine where a child is in their overall development.

2. Reflex-specific tests: Each primitive reflex has a specific test designed to elicit the reflex response. For example, to test the ATNR, the evaluator may ask the child to turn their head to one side while lying down, and then observe the position of their limbs. Similarly, to assess the Moro reflex, the evaluator may simulate a sudden drop or use a sudden loud noise to provoke a response. Each reflex has its unique test, and the professional will carefully observe the child's reactions. This is the easiest and most used way to determine if a reflex is present.

3. Standardized assessments: Some professionals use standardized assessments to evaluate primitive reflexes and overall motor development. These assessments such as the Peabody Developmental Motor Scales, the Bruininks–Oseretsky Test of Motor Proficiency, or the Movement Assessment Battery for Children can help determine if a child's motor skills are age-appropriate and identify potential concerns.

4. Sensory processing evaluation: Because retained primitive reflexes can affect a child's sensory processing, professionals may use sensory processing evaluations to assess how a child responds to different sensory inputs. The Sensory Profile or the Sensory Integration and Praxis Tests are examples of tools used to evaluate sensory processing.

5. Parental input and questionnaires: Parental observations and input are invaluable in assessing primitive reflexes. Professionals may ask parents to complete questionnaires or provide detailed information about their child's behavior, developmental milestones, and any other concerns they have. This information can help the evaluator better understand the child's overall development and guide the assessment process.

6. Medical history and examination: A thorough medical history and physical examination are essential components of the assessment process. The professional will gather information about the child's birth, developmental milestones, and any medical issues that might be relevant to their motor development. A physical examination can help rule out any underlying medical conditions that might be contributing to the child's difficulties.

It is important to note that assessment techniques and tools may vary depending on the professional's expertise and the child's specific needs. After completing the evaluation, the professional will provide a diagnosis, discuss the findings with the parents, and recommend appropriate interventions and support to address any retained primitive reflexes and their impact on the child's development.

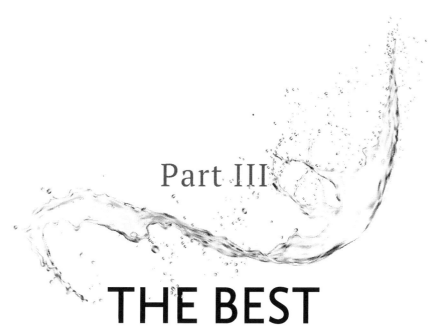

Part III

THE BEST
INTERVENTION

THE MAGIC OF INTENSIVES

As we have described previously, primitive reflexes originate in various regions of the brain. If a reflex persists, it indicates that the reflex is present in an attempt to stimulate the corresponding area of the brain and aid in its development. Engaging in activities that strengthen these brain areas is crucial to efficiently and effectively eliminate these reflexes. Each area of the brain can be targeted with specific activities to enhance its strength. Once this is accomplished, the reflex will naturally fade away.

Before studying functional neurology, I held the belief that repetitive movements had to be performed hundreds or even thousands of times to provide the brain with sensory input and facilitate integration, leading to the elimination of primitive reflexes. However, I discovered that by specifically activating and stimulating the weak areas and hemispheres of the brain through different exercises or modalities, the reflexes can disappear much more rapidly on their own. In many cases, reflexes vanish within minutes, although the duration of intervention required can vary from one week to six weeks, depending on the intensity of the approach employed.

As I continued to learn about functional neurology, the appointments became longer and longer. Today, I refer to these long appointments as "intensives." Today, I see patients from all over the country and the world for intensives, which consist of two to four hours of therapy per day for one to four weeks at a time. In just a week or two, retained reflexes can often become integrated. This model of care has wholly revolutionized my office and enabled me to help patients I could never help before.

With the right amounts and kinds of stimulation, oxygen, and energy, the brain can function properly, and retained reflexes can integrate quickly and effectively. I refer to stimulation, oxygen, and energy as the brain development trifecta.

STIMULATION, OXYGEN, AND ENERGY

The intensive model capitalizes on this trifecta; we make sure our patients get enough stimulation, oxygen, and energy in the appropriate sequence to support brain energy metabolism. This brain energy metabolism results in the formation of adenosine triphosphate (ATP), which is essential for maintaining basic electrophysiological activities in a "resting" brain and supporting evoked neuronal activity when the brain is active. Such activities are crucial for overall brain growth, connectivity, and development, including the integration of primitive reflexes.

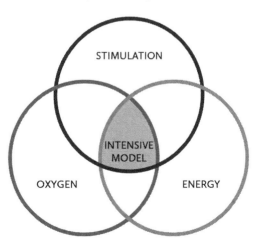

Stimulation

Stimulating weak or underdeveloped brain areas assists with brain development. Hence, in our initial physical examination, we identify these weaknesses or underdeveloped regions. While working on primitive reflexes, we can also stimulate the midline cerebellum, which coordinates balance; the frontal lobe, which coordinates attentional networks; or the parietal lobe, which gives us sensory perception. Doing this allows the brain to better regulate these reflexes and to coordinate the balance centers and eyes more appropriately.

Oxygen

Getting oxygen to the system is simple. We monitor a child's oxygen saturation during therapy. If their oxygen saturation starts to drop, we make sure they have enough oxygen for their system. If their oxygen goes down and their heart rate goes up, indicating their system is fatigued and doesn't have enough oxygen, we can provide supplemental oxygen. We also use exercise with oxygen therapy at times, allowing us to get more oxygen to the system because a person exercising produces much more carbon dioxide. As carbon dioxide increases in the system, the body can absorb more oxygen. Depending on a child's condition or injury, we may also hook them up to an oxygen concentrator if needed.

We also use hyperbaric oxygen therapy. This is an excellent tool before or after physical rehab. We put the patient in a large, soft chamber and then pressurize the chamber. Putting pressure behind oxygen forces it deeper into our tissues, so as pressure rises, oxygen is pushed into our cells. When we push oxygen into a cell or mitochondria, we can produce more ATP. The more energy our cells have, the better they can do their job, and the brain and body can develop and function.

Energy

Energy is essential to overall health and development. At the cellular level, ATP is our source of energy and enables a person's cells to function. Furthermore, ATP can only be produced if the cell's mitochondria are functioning properly.

Research indicates that laser light therapy can improve mitochondrial function, stem cell function, connectivity, and neuron migration. However, research also indicates that simple things like food dyes can prevent the mitochondria from functioning properly. It is vital that parents begin and continue to nourish their children while they grow, undergo intensives, and integrate primitive reflexes.

MAXIMIZING INTENSIVES

Even though we have fantastic tools at the office to allow us to get more oxygen and produce more energy, parents must ensure their children receive a healthy diet and live in a safe, supportive environment that fosters their children's growth, development, and long-term success.

Low-Carb, High Fat, Adequate Protein Diet

Eating a balanced diet of macronutrients (fat, protein, and carbohydrates) is important for health. Fat is the macronutrient with the most ATP production, so consuming healthy fats can help maximize the effectiveness of intensives. Gram for gram, sugar produces much less ATP than healthy fats, so when kids are on a diet high in carbohydrates, they often experience energy deficiency. Similarly, a diet of highly processed carbohydrates can also lead to energy deficiency because it lacks the vitamins and minerals cells need to function properly. When mitochondria and other organelles in the cells don't function properly, less ATP is produced.

Ensuring your child is on a low-carb, high-fat, and adequate protein diet before, during, and after intensives greatly benefits brain development. I suggest feeding your child a paleo diet because it contains adequate fat, vegetables, and antioxidants. I also recommend getting rid of highly processed carbs that lack nutritional value and can create gut issues. Avoiding high-inflammatory foods such as gluten and dairy and consuming nutrient-dense foods such as vegetables, healthy meats, and healthy fats will build a system that can mature and develop efficiently.

When you eat, you are literally feeding your cells, gut, and brain. An array of colorful fruits and vegetables provide the vitamins, minerals, and antioxidants your cells need to make ATP. They also provide the gut with the fiber it needs to process and digest food well. As mentioned earlier, the brain uses fat efficiently for fuel, also relying on cholesterol and fat for proper nerve connection. Finally, people (especially children) need adequate protein because protein serves as the building blocks for the body. Ensuring food is "clean" is important; grass-fed and organic sources are ideal.

Diets that are gluten-free, dairy-free, and low in sugar (e.g., paleo diets) are especially beneficial for children with neurodevelopmental delays because they limit inflammation in the brain, sinuses, and body. Large blood sugar swings in children have been shown to accompany brain fog, behavioral outbursts, energy decline, and attention problems. The presence of healthy fats and proteins in their diets can help these children regulate their energy more consistently and efficiently.

What about supplements? Well, it is important to remember that supplements are only "supplemental," and that no supplement in the world can replace a healthy diet. Many supplements are synthetic, even the good-quality ones, and our bodies can't process them as well. That said, I sometimes recommend the following supplements because they help limit inflammation and promote gut health:

1. Omega-3 fish oils
2. Probiotics
3. Methylated B vitamins
4. Whole-food vitamin C

All in all, a poor diet is like putting the cheapest gas in your car; it's going to burn quickly. A nutritious diet low in sugar and dense in fruits, vegetables, healthy fats, and protein is like putting premium fuel in your car; it will burn cleaner and much more efficiently.

Clean Home Environment

A clean home environment includes clean food and is free from chemicals and toxins. The fewer toxins in our everyday lives, the less stress there is on our body. The less stress there is on the body, the more likely we are to develop properly. The toxins that disrupt proper development, especially in children, include the following items:

- Mold
- Chemicals in cleaning and personal care products
- Plastic serving and storage containers
- Drinking or bathing in tap water
- Teflon dishes or pans
- Fluoride toothpaste
- Fluorescent lights

These toxins can build up in a child's body and hinder their ability to detoxify and develop. Removing any mold, using "clean" household and personal care products, storing food in glass containers rather than plastic, changing your furnace filters consistently, adding Air Doctor air purifiers, installing a water filtration system, cooking with safe dishes and pans, and using non-fluoride toothpaste can help create a cleaner home environment for the whole family.

Minimizing screen time as much as possible is also important. Instead of screens, children need physical activity, fresh air, and good old-fashioned playtime so they can develop a healthy lung capacity, cardiovascular system, and brain.

LET IT RAIN, FLOOD THE BRAIN, AND REST

Importance of Rain and Flooding the Brain

Years of clinical experience have shown that using an intensive model combined with a nutritious diet and healthy environment is the best way to facilitate brain development. In a standard care model, it takes six to eighteen months to integrate primitive reflexes because children only get fifteen minutes of therapy three times a week. I can confidently say that the intensive method is far superior. By working intensely with children (two to four hours per day for one to two weeks at a time), helping parents through diet and environment improvements, and allowing adequate time between intensives, children can make incredible progress.

Envision the brain's pathways as a river. When you get a lot of rain, that river gets bigger and bigger. In the brain, think of that rain as a stimulus. When we stimulate the brain or get more rain, the river gets larger and larger, allowing for better and more robust pathways. We activate those pathways, and more and more connections form as a result.

If that river gets big enough, it continues flowing for several months without rain. In the same way, if we can see those patients for a more extended period and give them enough stimulus, they'll begin using their brain and body differently, forming new pathways. When we do that for many days, those pathways remain strong and continue developing even after the patient returns home. We can change the brain by doing this, but it can take a lot of stimuli to kick-start the process. In essence, we should "let it rain" and "flood the brain" with stimulus up front so that the brain can integrate the primitive reflexes and establish new pathways necessary for reading, learning, and living as well as overall growth, strength, health, and healing.

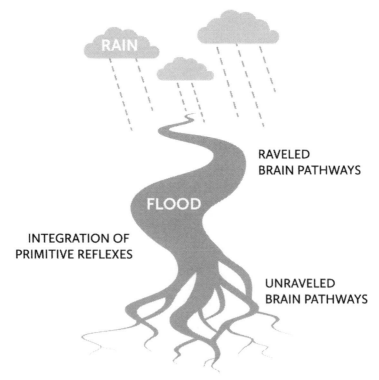

RAIN

RAVELED
BRAIN PATHWAYS

FLOOD

INTEGRATION OF
PRIMITIVE REFLEXES

UNRAVELED
BRAIN PATHWAYS

IMPROVEMENTS IN READING, LEARNING, AND LIVING

Importance of Rest and Recovery

When I ran track at a high level, we used training cycles to increase our performance. We'd do two to three weeks of challenging workouts, followed by a week of rest and recovery, and then another two to three weeks of intense workouts, followed by another week of rest and recovery.

During the intense weeks, we worked hard under a heavy load, and our bodies responded by maturing and increasing capacity. But after a week of rest, we were stronger and faster than when training hard. Why is this? Our bodies need time to rest and recover between intense training sessions. The brain is no different. It can quickly create neuroplasticity and synapses but craves rest to develop and recover.

I believe this adds to the magic of the intensive model. When someone comes in for a week or two straight, we work with them intensely. Then we send them home with tools and exercises to work on that are less intense, but they reinforce what we did in the office and keep those neural pathways firing. Then they may come back a few weeks or months later for another round of intense therapy. Using this method, I see almost unbelievable changes in developmentally challenged children whom I'm unable to help using the traditional model of care.

Capitalizing on Neuroplasticity

Intensives capitalize on something known as neuroplasticity, or brain plasticity. This is the ability of neural networks in the brain to change through reorganization and growth. This change or rewiring allows the brain to function differently than previously. During intensives, we strive for as much reorganization as possible. When the patient goes home, we then set up a program that facilitates as much growth as possible. This growth allows the patient's body to adapt, change, and use muscles differently. This growth also allows the brain and body to work better together. As a result, a child's movement, balance, and hand–eye coordination all improve.

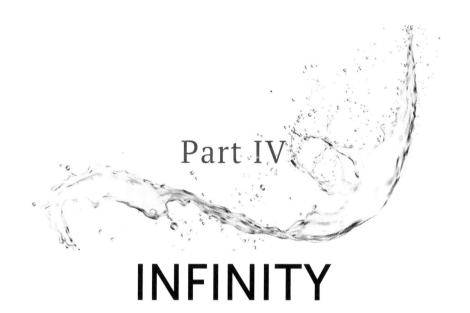

Part IV

INFINITY

OPEN INVITATION

We realize that our clinic and intensives may not be for everyone. Maybe you have a doctor you're satisfied with already. Maybe the logistics of traveling to Iowa or one of the clinics does not work for your family schedule or budget. But if you're willing and able to invest in an intensive, please call or stop by our clinic anytime. By working with our amazing team and proven model, I guarantee your child can make major strides in their ability to read, learn, and live. I know this because children arrive daily at Infinity Functional Neurology with severe challenges and leave one or two weeks later having made excellent progress. Let me introduce you to some of them.

SUCCESS STORIES

"Blake"

I first realized intensives could make a massive difference quickly while working with one of the first patients who came to see me from far away. At that point, I was using a more traditional care model, but people from out of state began asking for a way to work with me, too. I knew that nonlocal patients couldn't see me two times a week for three months, so I had them come for one to two weeks instead and worked with them for several hours per day to maximize their time in the office.

One of the first kids I saw using this method came from Chicago. We'll call him Blake. Blake's parents brought him to me to see if I could help with his learning and reading issues. He had many struggles in the classroom, but the main problem was that he was in fourth grade but barely reading at a first-grade level. Despite having multiple tutors, he couldn't catch up. His parents didn't know what to do, so they brought him to me.

I found that Blake had many nonintegrated primitive reflexes. His balance systems weren't well-developed, and his eyes couldn't track or work together appropriately. These foundational issues needed correcting for learning to occur, so we got to work.

With this child, the intensive method was the only approach that could've helped him because he had many abnormal movement patterns from using his primitive reflexes for so long. It was wild to observe his movements when he first arrived at the office. If I moved his right hand, the whole left side of his body moved. If I moved his right foot, his head began rotating in the opposite direction. When primitive reflexes are retained past the age they should integrate, I observe significant abnormal reflexive movement.

In this young man's case, his eyes began jumping around when he tried reading a book, and his body began moving through reflexive activation. He couldn't control or stop it. Think of trying to read, but your eyes can't track the line of text, and your body jumps all over the place.

No wonder Blake was struggling.

During the first intensive, we retrained his reflexes by slowly retraining his range of motion. It took me three days having him lie on his back and move all his extremities and the whole body slowly to retrain his motor movements, so he didn't have quick, reflexive activation in his muscles. Over several days, his primitive reflexes integrated and went away. That was the only thing we accomplished during the first intensive. He came back about eight weeks later. By then, he was reading at a fourth-grade level, which was truly remarkable. He hadn't fully caught up to his peers, but he was much closer simply because we had integrated his reflexes.

During his second intensive, we focused on rehabilitating his vestibular system, stabilizing his eyes, and tracking his eyes appropriately. Within another week, we were able to accomplish these goals. I haven't seen this young man since the end of his second intensive because his reading has improved so much. He's now at grade level in all skills, growing and maturing as he should. His parents are thrilled and tell me he's doing extremely well.

The intensive method is why my team and I helped this young man make such massive gains in only two weeks in the office. If I had seen that child for thirty minutes twice a week for three months, I wouldn't have been able to get close to the same results. I know this because I've done it the traditional way. Yet we're constantly learning, growing, adapting, and making new processes as we see more and more patients and help them attain better results. If I had seen this young man a year earlier before I was using the intensive method, or if he'd been a local patient, the results wouldn't have been comparable.

"Kyle"

Kyle had a diagnosis of Down syndrome and autism. His parents brought him to me because he was constantly stimming— self-stimulating repetitive or unusual body movement or noises. He couldn't learn anything new or improve his skills of any kind because he couldn't stop stimming. It was all he did for hours on end.

We used the intensive method with him because he was from far away. His parents brought him to our office for two weeks straight, and we worked with him for two hours daily— the maximum amount of time he could handle. Providing his brain enough activation and stimulus through the methods and technology we use in the office was difficult because he constantly moved. Any light, sound, or vibration on his body caused significant movement reactions. However, we slowly and methodically introduced the stimulation and got him to a point where he began calming down. Once that happened, we started working on integrating his primitive reflexes. By the end of his two-week intensive, he could sit, stand, and follow simple directions. His stimming dramatically decreased to where he was only doing it minimally throughout the day. He also began making eye contact, playing with toys, and connecting with his siblings. He even tried verbalizing. His words weren't understandable, but he tried, which he'd never done before. He became much more aware of his surroundings and began pointing at objects. Before coming to the office, his parents said he didn't do anything besides stim.

Again, if we hadn't done the intensive method with him and hadn't taken all that time to activate his brain, we wouldn't have seen dramatic changes. If we would've done a traditional model of care, there's no way we'd have helped him make those significant changes. The intensive method applied over a couple of weeks was what his brain needed to mature and develop.

Kyle returned for a second intensive, and working with him the second time was a completely different experience. He was able to do almost everything we asked him to do. He was no longer stimming. We had another impactful session and made tremendous progress.

"Sam"

Sam fell off the back of a truck and sustained a severe traumatic brain injury. He actually died during the accident and then came back to life. Doctors told him he would never function normally or move his body appropriately again.

When he first came to my office, I only did fifteen-minute appointments. But with him, I did three one-hour sessions per week. He was one of my first experiences with a more intensive model of care because I knew he had severe brain injury and needed as much time as I could give him if he were to have any hope of healing.

When Sam first began coming for therapy, he barely spoke except to yell profanities. His brain injury was that severe. I used many different tools to help him, including hyperbaric oxygen therapy, primitive reflex remediation, and lasers to calm inflammation. After six months of treatment in our office, his primitive reflexes were integrated, his eyes were moving and tracking appropriately, and his brain healed to the point where he could walk normally. Today, he's a college sophomore earning straight As. He drives back and forth to school and already has a job lined up after graduation.

Through much rehab and prayer, Sam's brain was restored to health. His story is another example of the power of the intensive method. With a traditional model of care, I wouldn't have had the time to utilize all the resources available in the office. But with the intensive method, we were able to make great strides toward helping him restore his health.

"Troy"

Like many other kids, Troy walked into our office wrestling with learning hurdles. Despite the label of dyslexia and substantial reading struggles, his spirit was undeterred. Unfortunately, Troy was falling behind his peers in school despite receiving specialized dyslexia tutoring. The tutoring sessions had become a point of pain and frustration for him, often leading him to question, "Why do you even take me to do this? It is torture." He would leave most sessions feeling defeated and hopeless.

When Troy came to us, we discovered several developmental issues that were impeding his progress. He had retained both asymmetrical and symmetrical tonic neck reflexes, inadequate development of his postural reflexes, and underdeveloped balance centers. His ability to track his eyes efficiently from side to side or up and down was compromised, and he struggled to converge his eyes well. Each of these challenges contributed to significant difficulties in his foundational learning abilities.

Nevertheless, Troy's journey didn't end there. After three months of targeted rehabilitation to address these deficits, a transformation began to take place. Troy, who once avoided reading, started finding joy in books. His dyslexia tutoring sessions turned from a source of despair into a platform for progress. He was rapidly closing the gap with his peers, nearly reaching grade level.

Troy's story is not one of a less capable child, but rather of a highly intelligent child who was missing some vital foundational skills needed for learning. With the right support and therapeutic interventions, Troy was able to overcome his learning challenges, reminding us all that each child has a unique path to success.

"Jenny"

A little girl came to the clinic with a rare genetic disorder that had made it difficult for her to crawl, and consequently she couldn't walk. A couple of weeks after her first intensive, her primitive reflexes had been integrated enough that she improved her motor coordination and took a total of twelve steps. Two months later, she came back for her second intensive. Her primitive reflexes seemed better, so we focused on her balance systems, including her vestibular systems. This allowed her to improve her balance, and she was able to take over twenty steps quite consistently. This type of progress is amazing, yet we see it every day.

We expect to see her progress continue at this rate as we work on the developmental sequence of her primitive reflexes. Until they are all integrated, we will continue to focus on her balance systems and then work on her vision, which will allow her to perform more and more functional activities and improve her quality of life.

Blake, Kyle, Sam, Troy, and Jenny are just a few of the children we've helped. We see children like them every day—children with rare genetic disorders, developmental delays, or traumatic brain injuries who go from being limited in life to becoming limitless in their capabilities. By simply walking them through the developmental blueprint, we changed their lives forever. Their lives became limitless.

GOOD IN ALL CIRCUMSTANCES

If you've made it to this part of the book, you probably have a child who has been struggling with behaviors, learning, and everyday life. Their life to date hasn't looked like you first imagined it to look, but let me encourage you. These struggles will be used for good!

When I was young, I was a lot like your child. I really struggled with reading, and even as a doctor, I still read at the rate of a fourth or fifth grader. I had reflexes and eye-tracking issues when I was young. I still have an eye convergence issue, and it's still challenging to keep my eyes stable when I'm reading. I forget what I'm reading if I read too fast.

I remember having multiple reading tutors. I remember not wanting to read in class because I was embarrassed. I remember being slower than everyone else and maybe peeking at my neighbor because I couldn't keep up. I remember not getting through my ACTs and having to put a C on half the test because I couldn't read the questions fast enough.

There were advantages to my struggles, though. I couldn't read fast, so I had to remember everything I read. My brain developed to the point where if I read something once, I remembered it for nearly forever. If I listen to something once, I remember it indefinitely. I can look at a page and remember it for a long time. I can see patterns in kids that most people can't see. A child with ADHD can come into the office, and I often immediately know what's going on because I've worked with so many of them. My brain can see the patterns. If I could read well and had good left brain function, I would not see patterns and solve problems in the same way. My right brain had to adapt and compensate, allowing me to do things others couldn't do.

I believe that God uses everything for good, including struggles. My struggles have prepared me to sympathize, empathize, understand, and serve children in ways few other medical professionals can. I wouldn't change my struggles for anything in the world.

Someday I hope you and your child will say the same thing. I would be honored to work with you and your child to make that happen. Together, we can make children be all God intended them to be: limitless!

ACKNOWLEDGMENTS

I want to thank all the doctors and medical professionals who came before me and set the foundations of functional neurology. I also want to thank my amazing staff for being so passionate about kids and for their willingness to grow and do whatever is necessary to help children reach their full potential.

ABOUT THE AUTHOR

Josh Madsen is a doctor of chiropractic, Fellow of the International Board of Functional Neurology, and co-owner of Infinity Functional Neurology. He is originally from Fort Dodge, Iowa, and received his undergraduate degree in exercise science from the University of Northern Iowa. He then became a doctor of chiropractic at Palmer College of Chiropractic. Dr. Josh also studied neurodevelopmental delays at the Carrick Institute of Clinical Neuroscience and rehabilitation and functional neurology at the Functional Neurology Seminars, accredited through the National University of Health Sciences. He is committed to equipping himself to better use functional neurology, chiropractic, and functional medicine to help children heal and have hope. He and his wife, Laryssa, have a son, James.

ABOUT THE COMPANY

Infinity helps children and adults with developmental delays, learning disabilities, and traumatic brain injuries. Dr. Josh and his ever-growing staff use chiropractic and functional neurology, a brain-based model, and the most current research and strategies to help parents and their children in their development. In a home-like environment, they test and assess patients' needs and goals and then create personalized plans to accomplish them. Using an "intensive" model of care where they spend two to four hours a day with a patient, Dr. Josh and his team of skilled, caring professionals capitalize on the time, tools, techniques, and technology required to help patients integrate primitive reflexes, grow, and make substantial progress in as little as a week or two—a fraction of the time usually required by a traditional model of care. After a strong neurological foundation is in place, patients leave the clinic and experience continual improvement in their everyday lives for weeks, months, and years to come. Infinity serves people from all fifty states and most continents and is committed to helping each patient achieve the best possible outcomes. Dr. Josh and his team are becoming known worldwide for their success in helping kids integrate primitive reflexes and transforming their ability to read, learn, and live.

Additional research and resources: LimitlessFoundation.co

Patient Resource Library:
https://www.iowainfinity.com/patient-resource-library

Contact Information
Infinity
95 NE Dartmoor Drive
Waukee, IA 50263
Office: (515) 264-3405
Website: https://www.iowainfinity.com
Facebook: https://www.facebook.com/infinityia/
Email: info@iowainfinity.com
Link Tree: linktr.ee/iowainfinity

Made in the USA
Monee, IL
12 October 2024

6b63c5d3-f7dc-4f7c-93db-2f9bc1b79235R01